The ABC's of Laughter

A
LAUGHTER DOODLES
Coloring Book
To Help You Make
an
Awesome Attitude Adjustment

by Sarah Routman

The ABC's of Laughter...

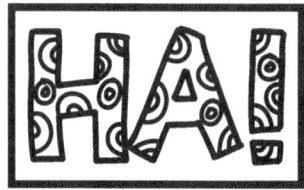
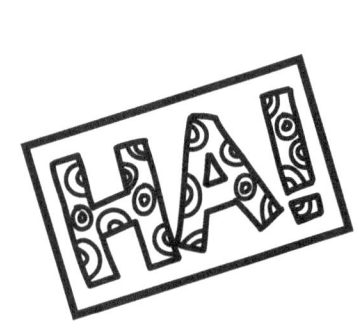
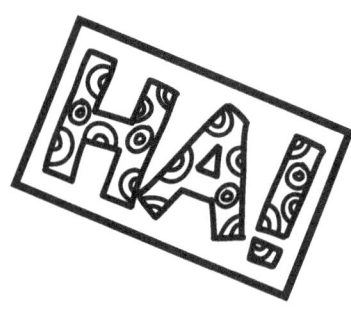

All the reasons you'll want to do it!

All the letters in this book can be sold as individual cards or pages.
Contact me for prints, cards or other images.
Sarah@LaughHealthy.com 612-802-1608
Find my photographs at
www.ThroughSarahsEyes.com

Laughter is serious business. Often misunderstood as something we do in reaction to something that is funny, Sarah's experience with Laughter Yoga has convinced her that there's more to giggles and guffaws than most people realize. Since your body doesn't know the difference between spontaneous and intentional laughter, giving you all the health benefits of laughter either way, why not put more laughter in *your* life, starting right now?!

Each letter in this book suggests a reason to laugh, but before you dig in to a glorious array of colors to grace the pages, consider these healthy benefits and try starting with gentle giggles as you color and then let go with wild abandon as you unleash a splash of color along with outrageous belly laughs! You won't believe the transformation that can happen.

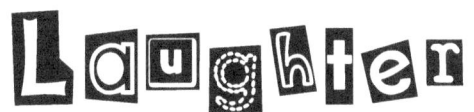

Decreases:	**Increases:**
Stress~Anxiety~Depression	Energy~Focus~Fun
Tension~Anger	Confidence~Calm
Nervousness~Boredom	Creativity
Pain	Positivity~Productivity
Blood Pressure	Oxygen to your cells

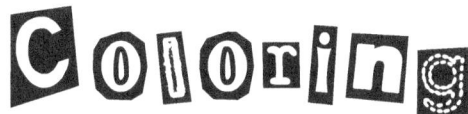

was prescribed by founder of analytical psychology, Carl Jung, to reduce anxiety and help patients become more centered and intentional as it boosts creativity and focus.

Grab your coloring tools, find a giggle in your pocket and discover the magic of letting laughter change your life!

Sarah Routman

LAUGHTER...

A is for **A**ll the reasons you'll want to do it!

to help you make an

Awesome

Attitude

Adjustment!

B -

B ecause it feels good...

C-

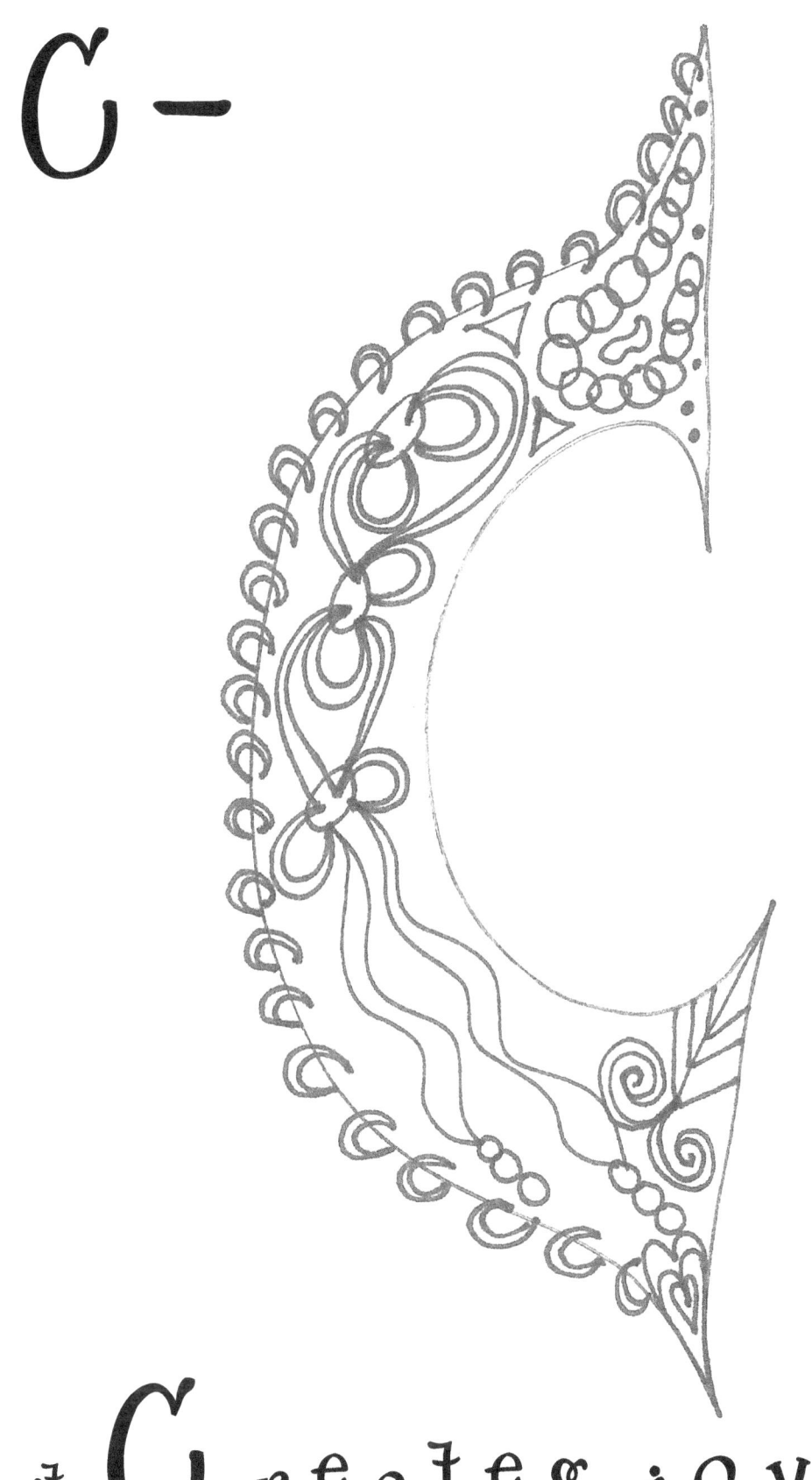

it Creates joy!

D-

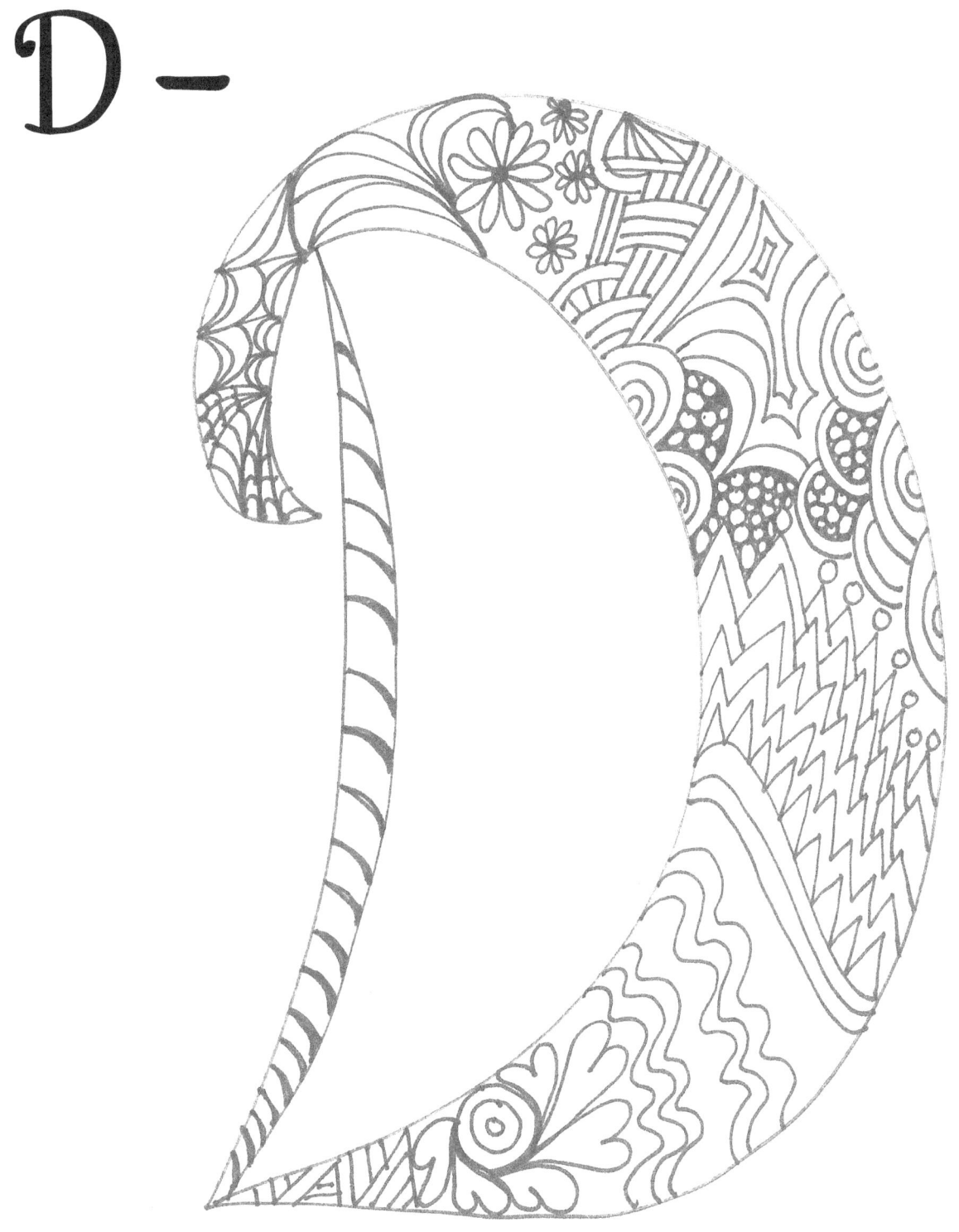

Do it Daily.

E -

E^{it} levates your mood.

E -

E [it] levates your mood.

F -

it's Fabulous FUN!

G-

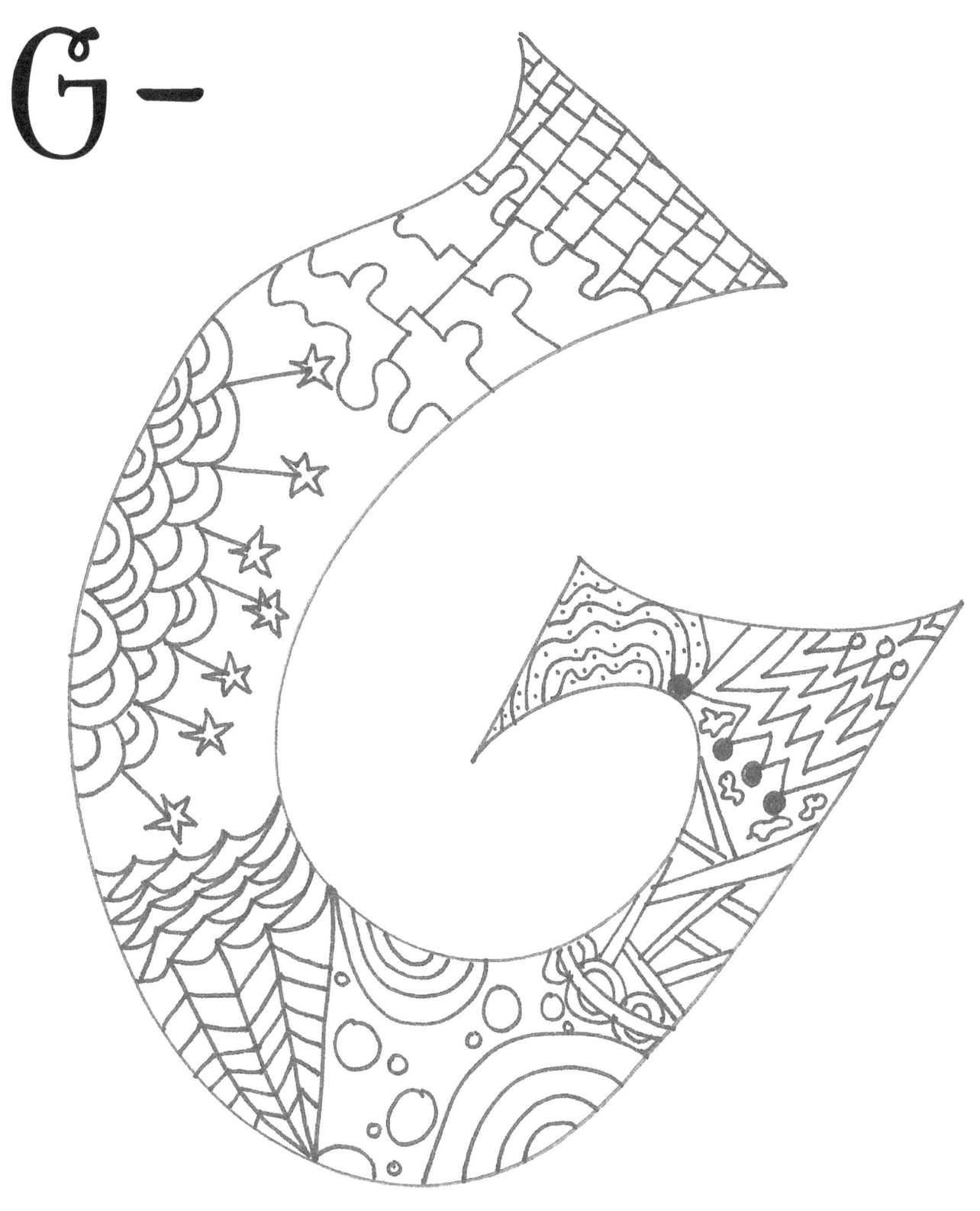

it's Great Exercise!

H —

it's Healthy.

i-

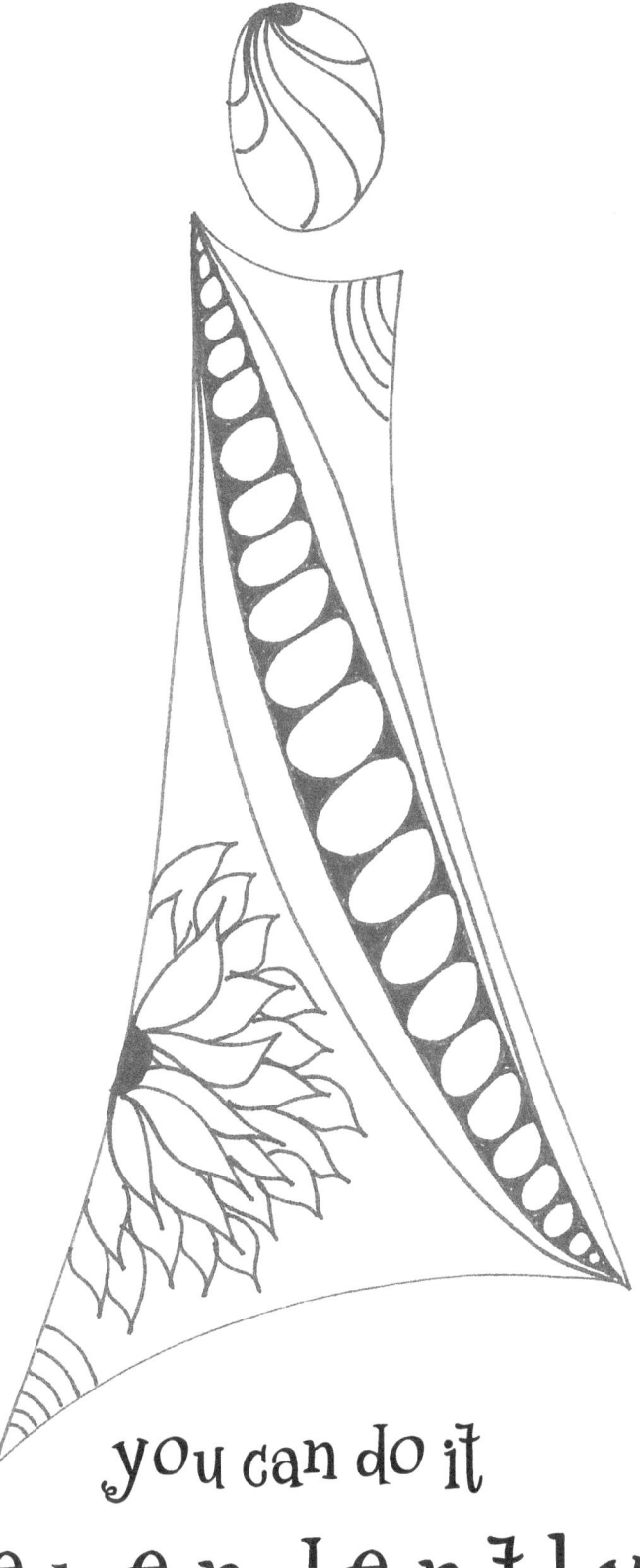

you can do it

Independently, or
with friends.

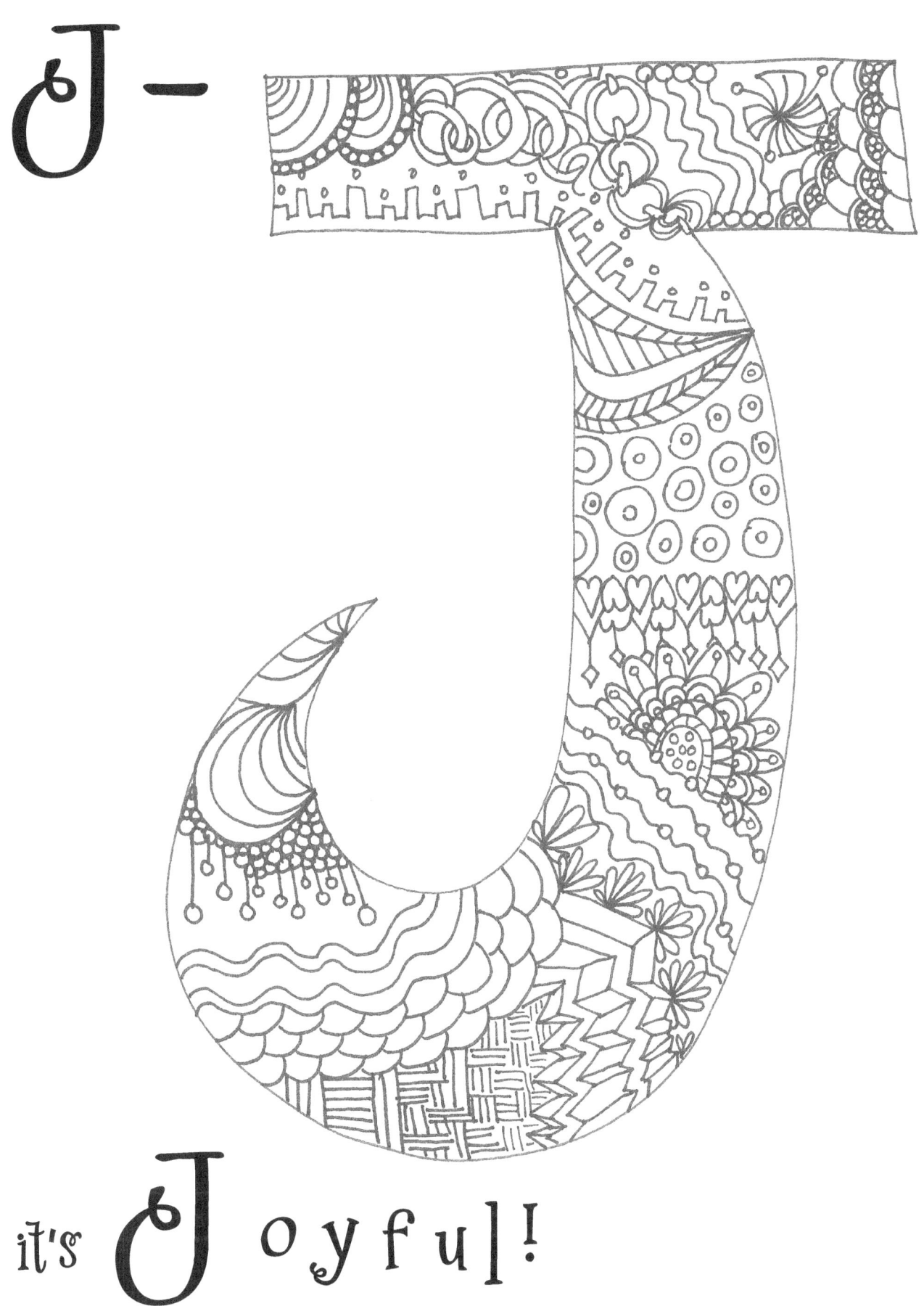

J –

it's **J**oyful!

K -

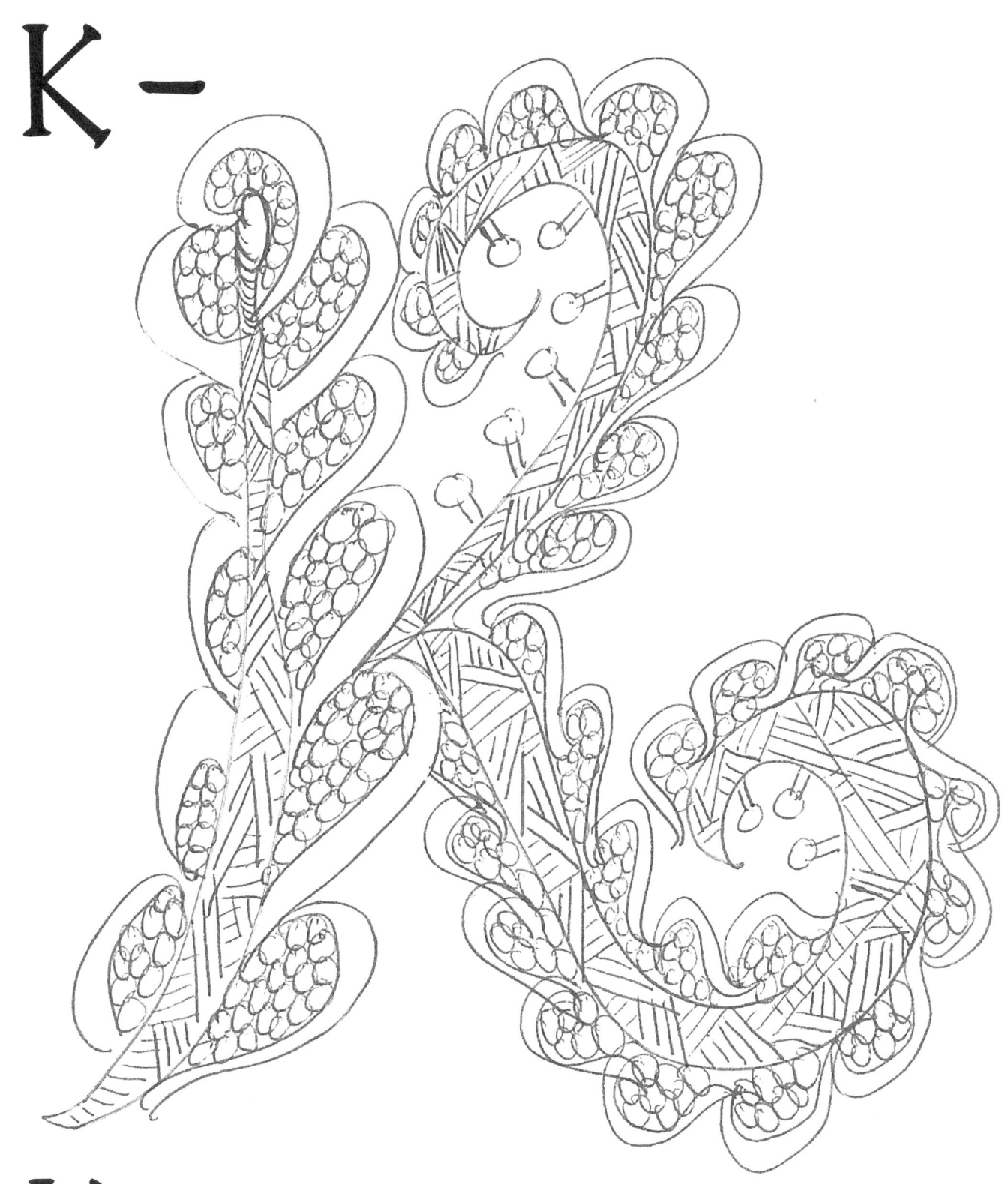

K eep doing it...

L -

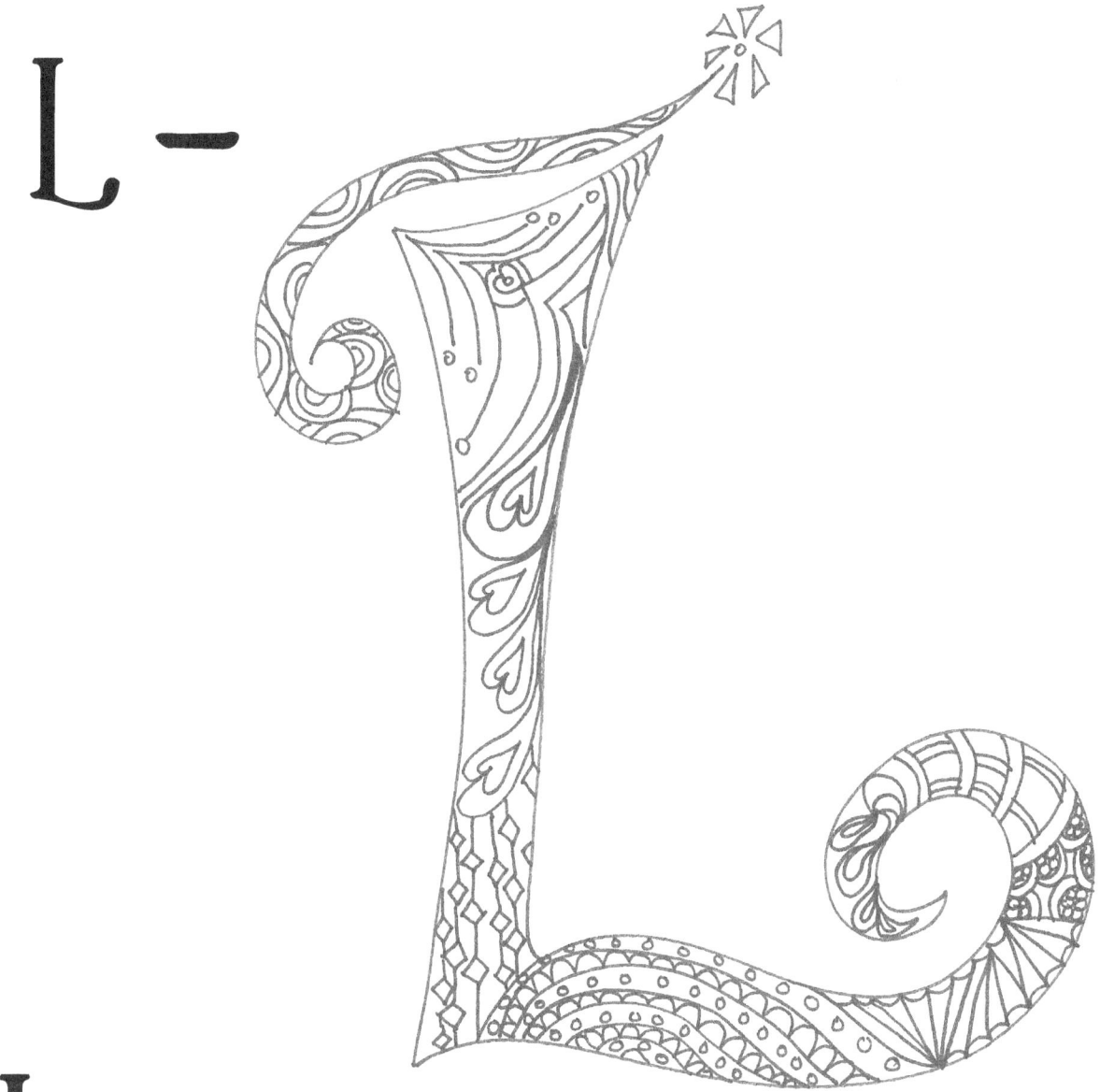

Lose weight with

Laughter and

Learn strategies to decrease stress.

M-

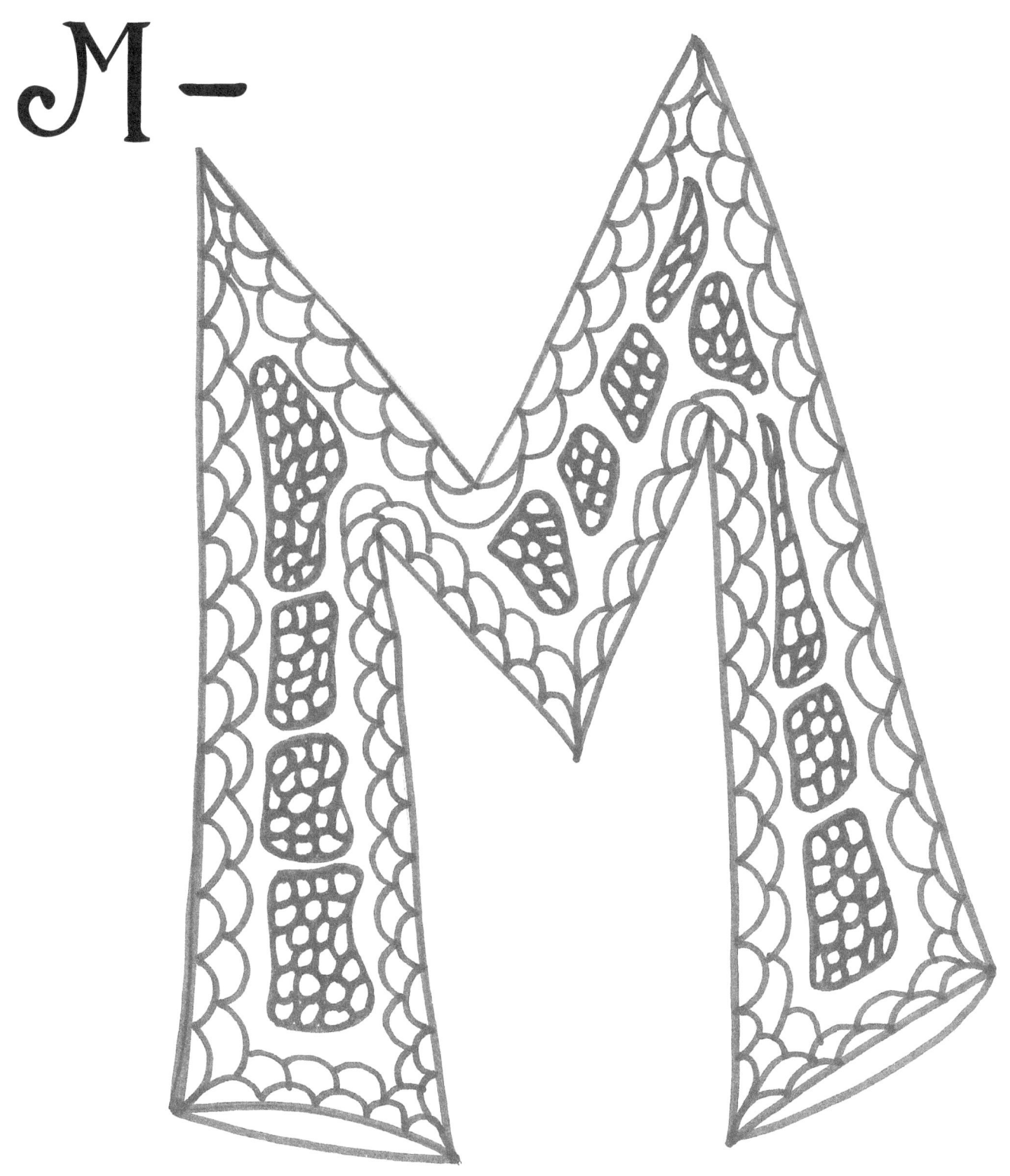

More is better.

n-

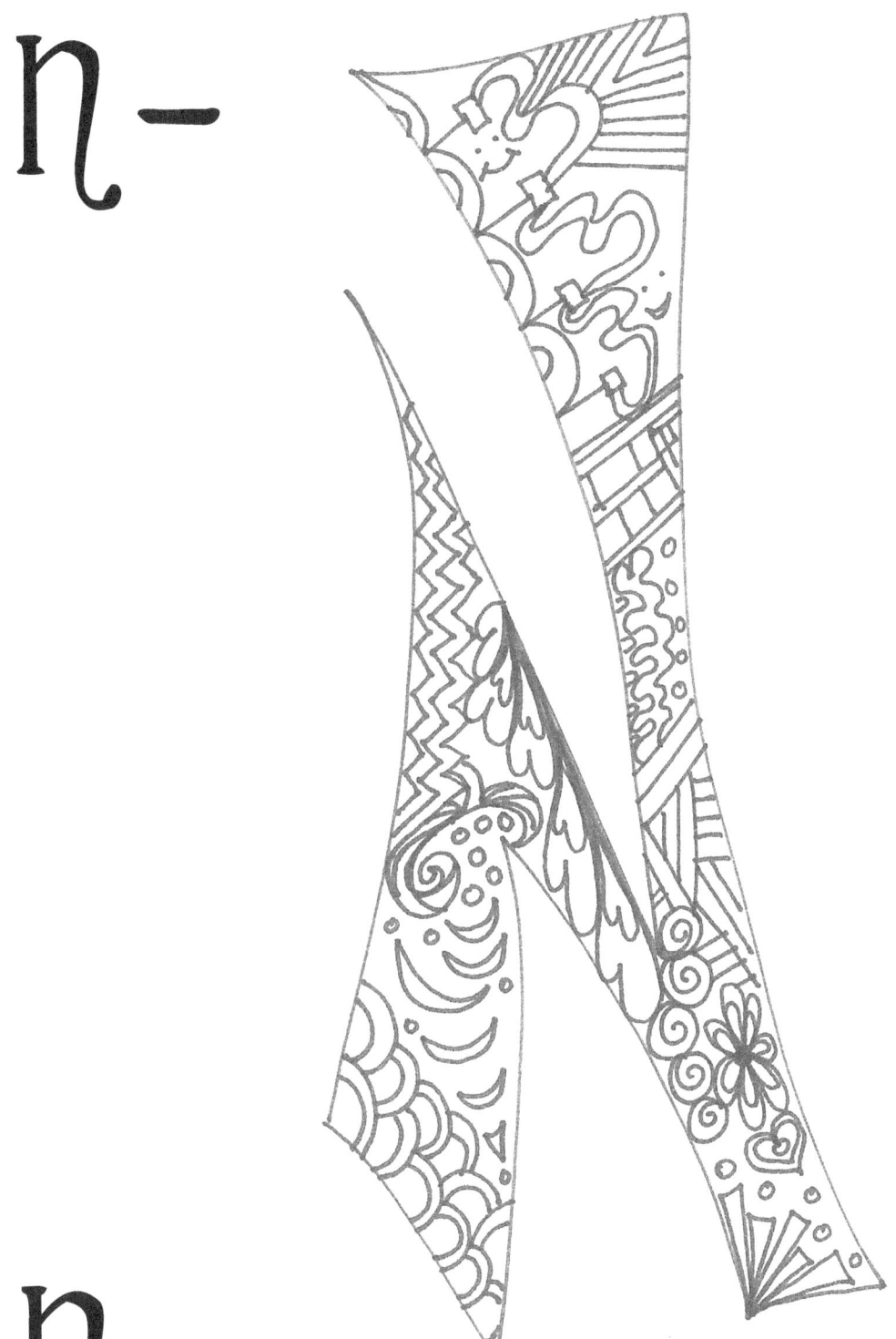

never underestimate the power of shared laughter.

O-

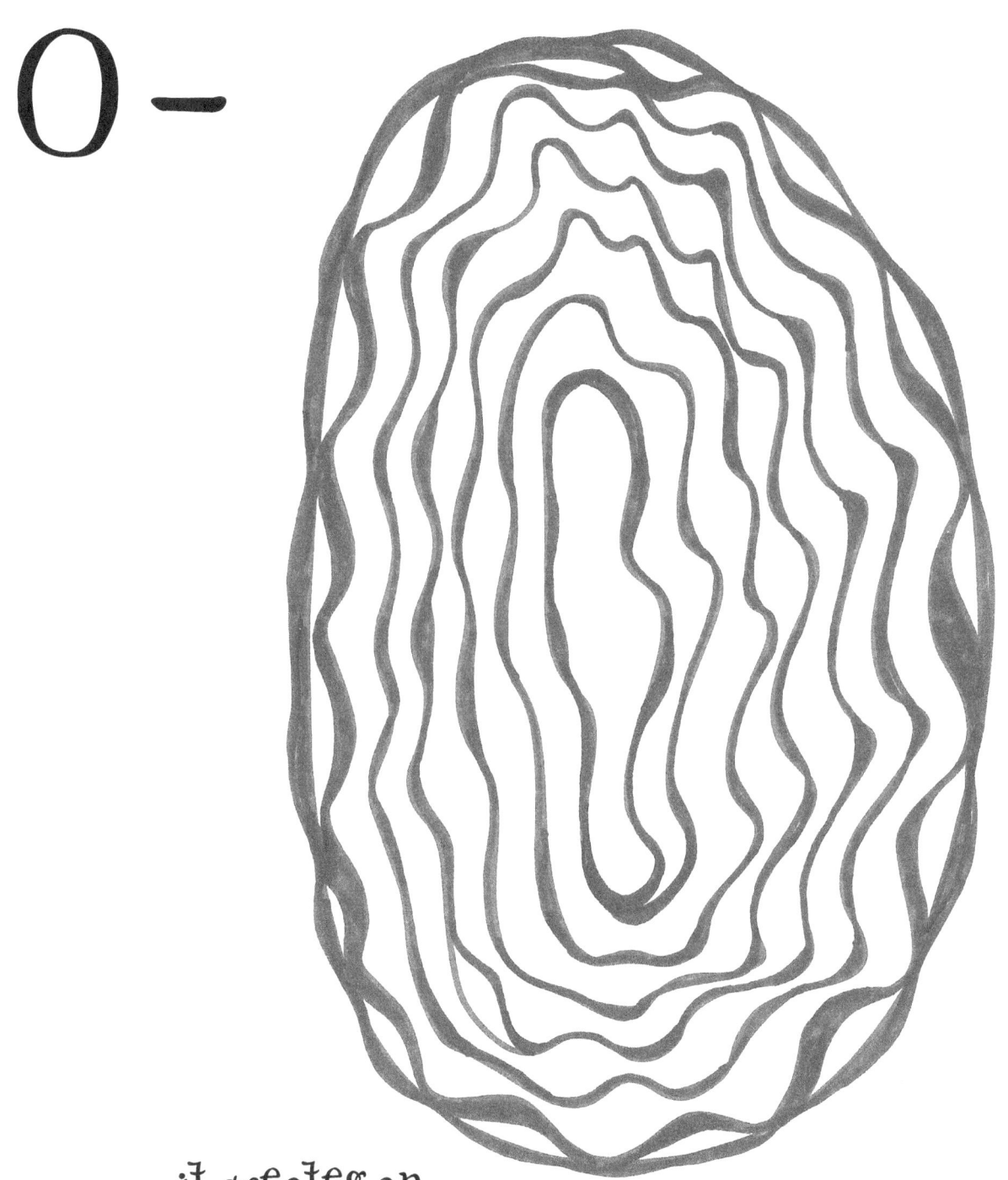

O

it creates an

pportunity for

O

penness.

P -

it's Playful and childlike.

Q -

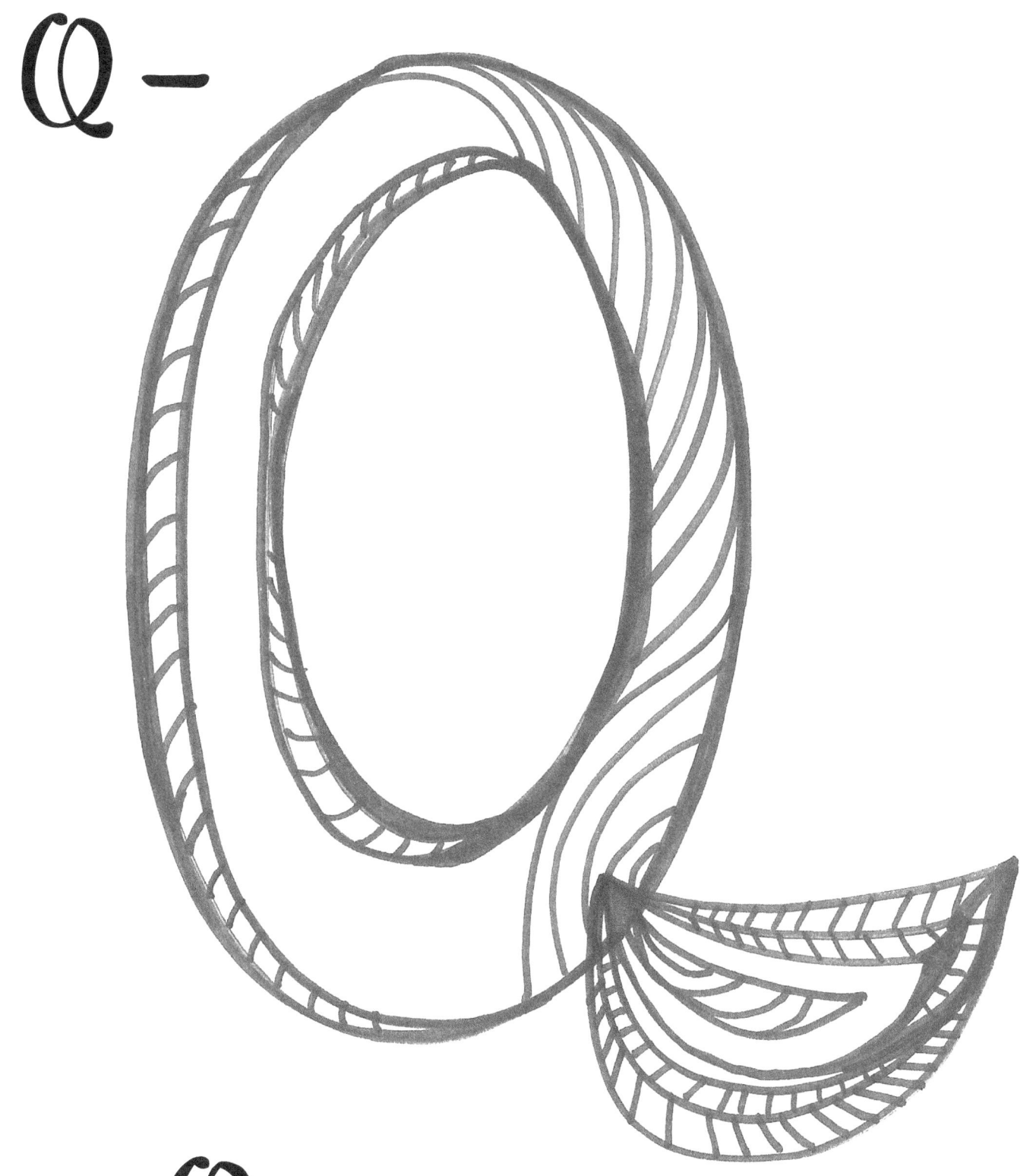

even Quiet laughter works.

R-

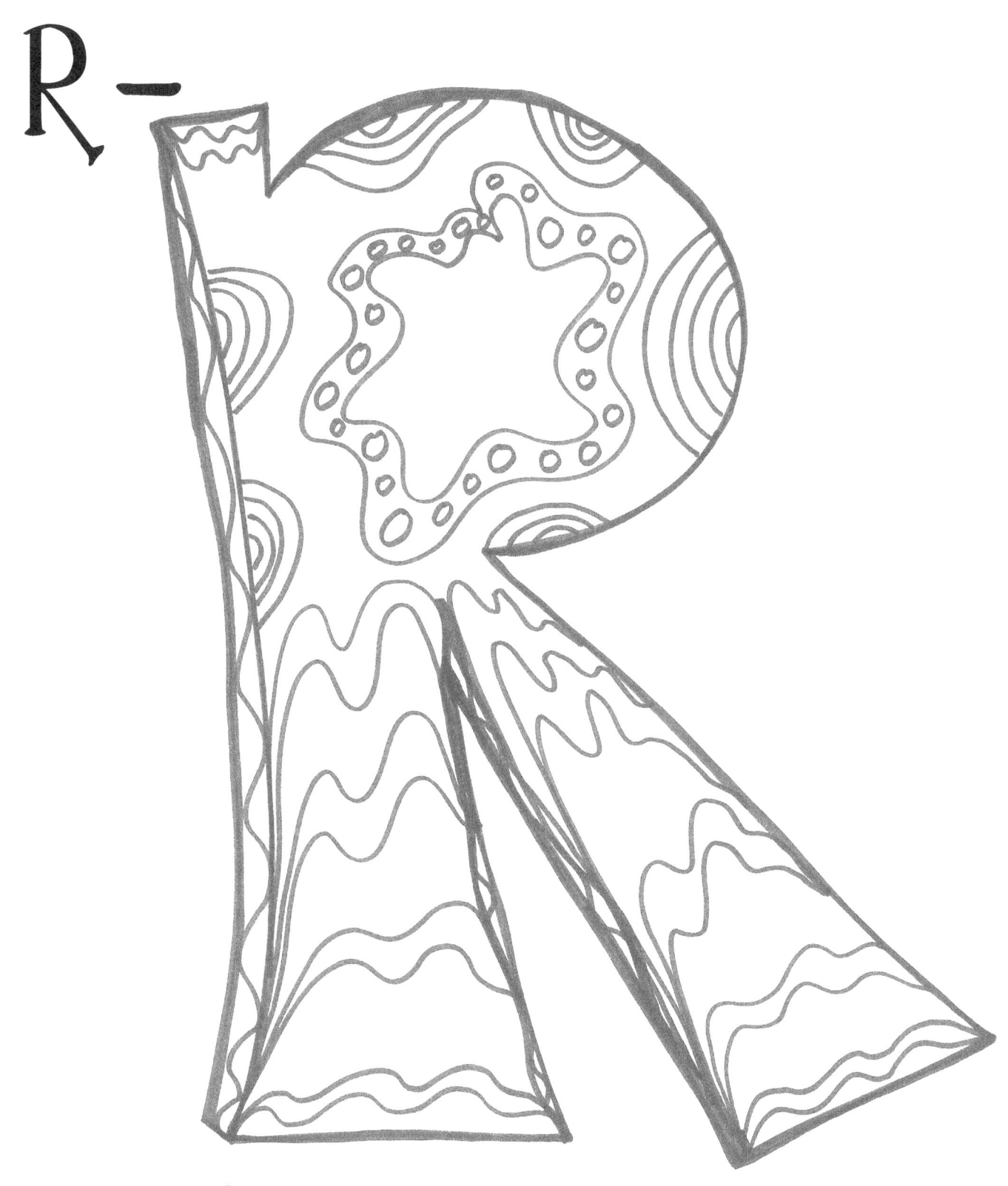

R it releases
Ridiculous FUN!

S -

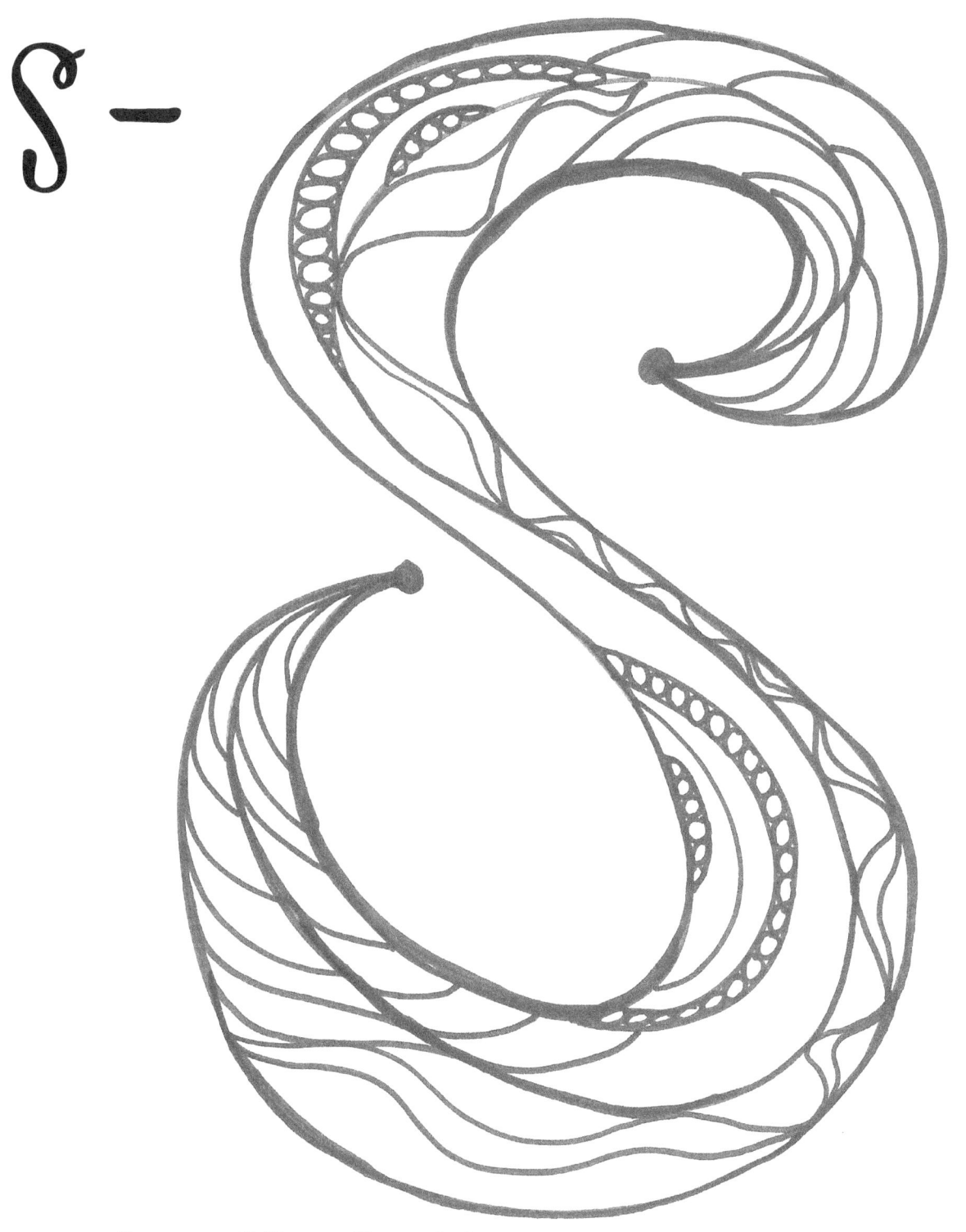

Laughter triggers
Serious Silliness!

T-

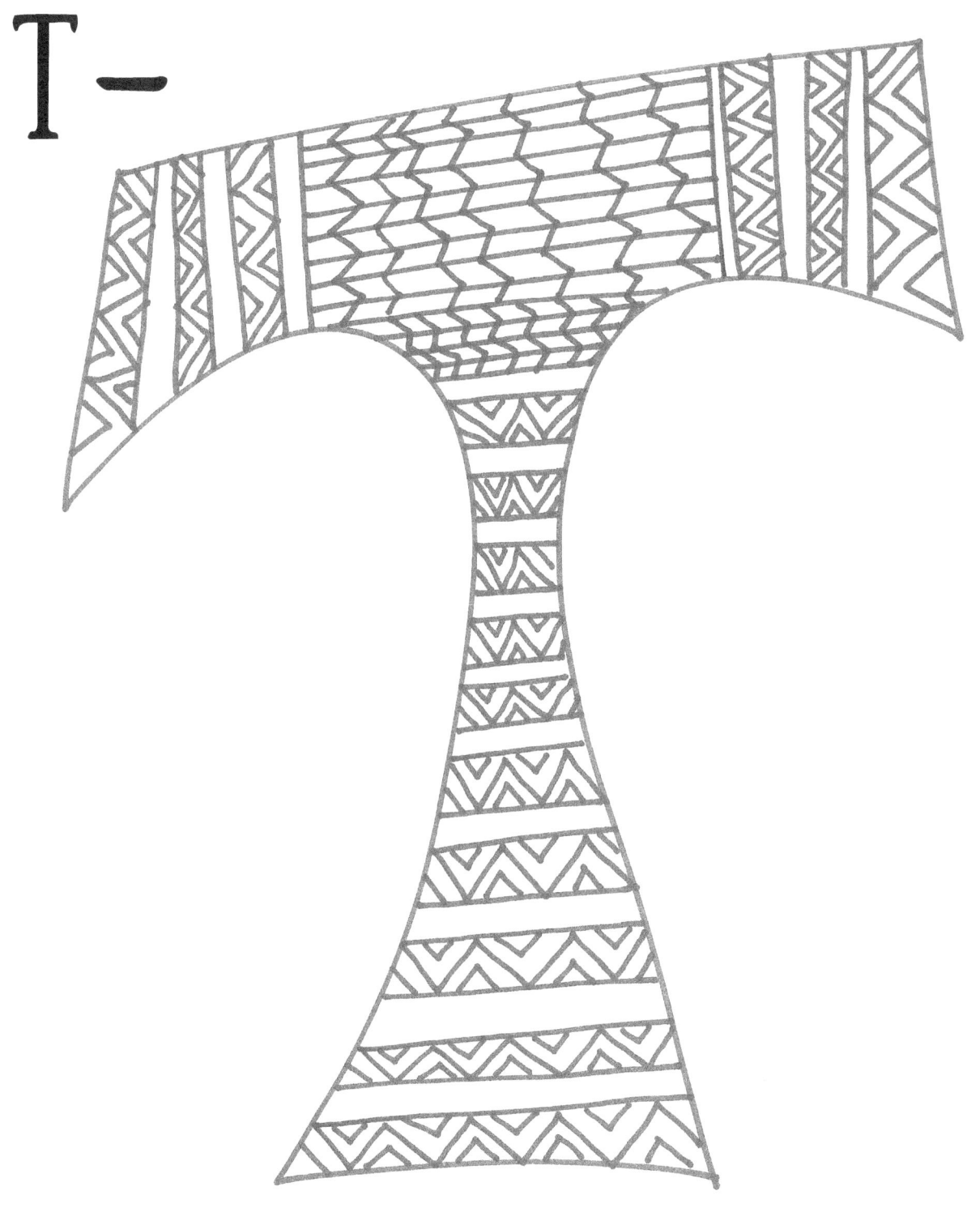

Take it with you
wherever you go.

U-

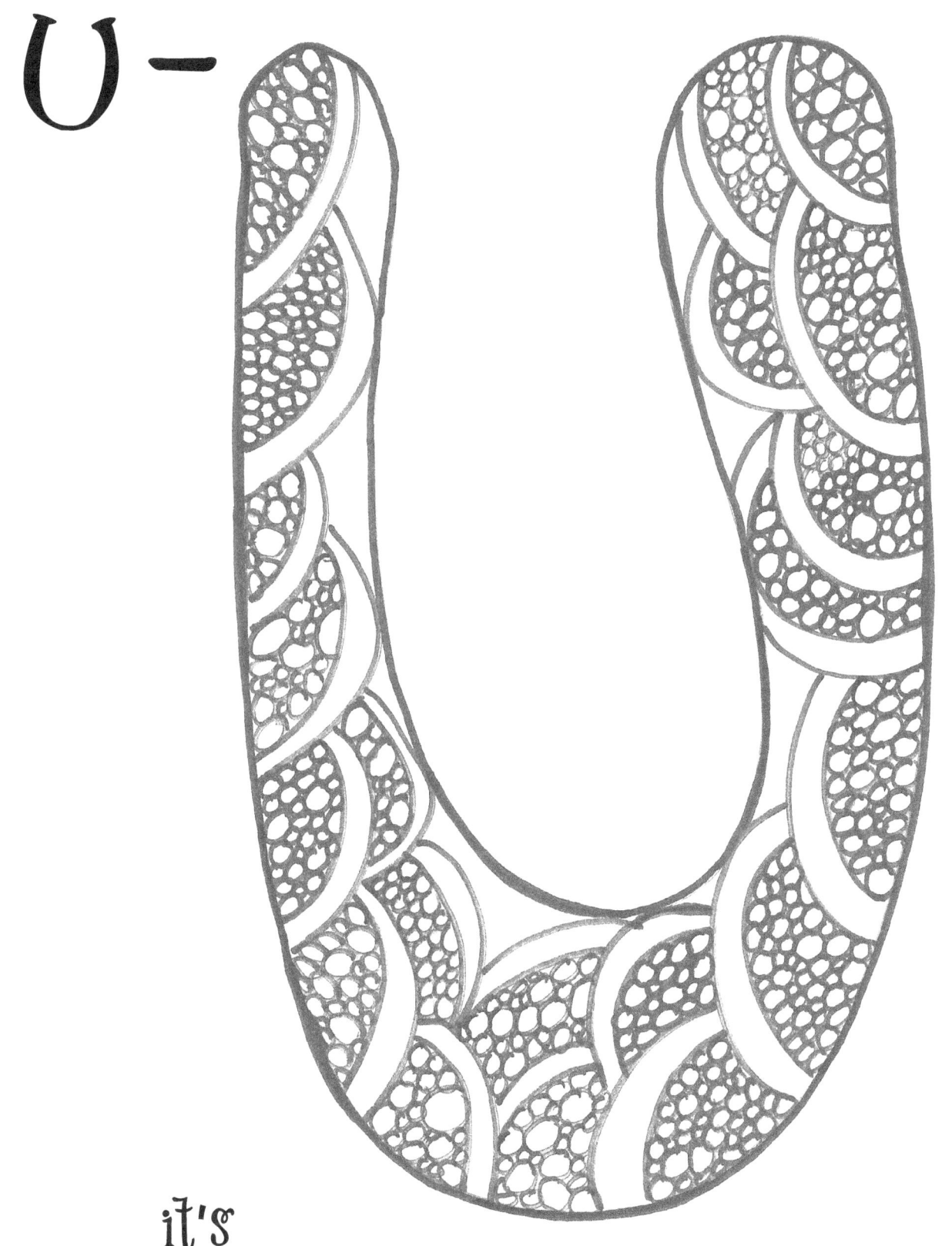

it's
Uniquely Uplifting!

V-

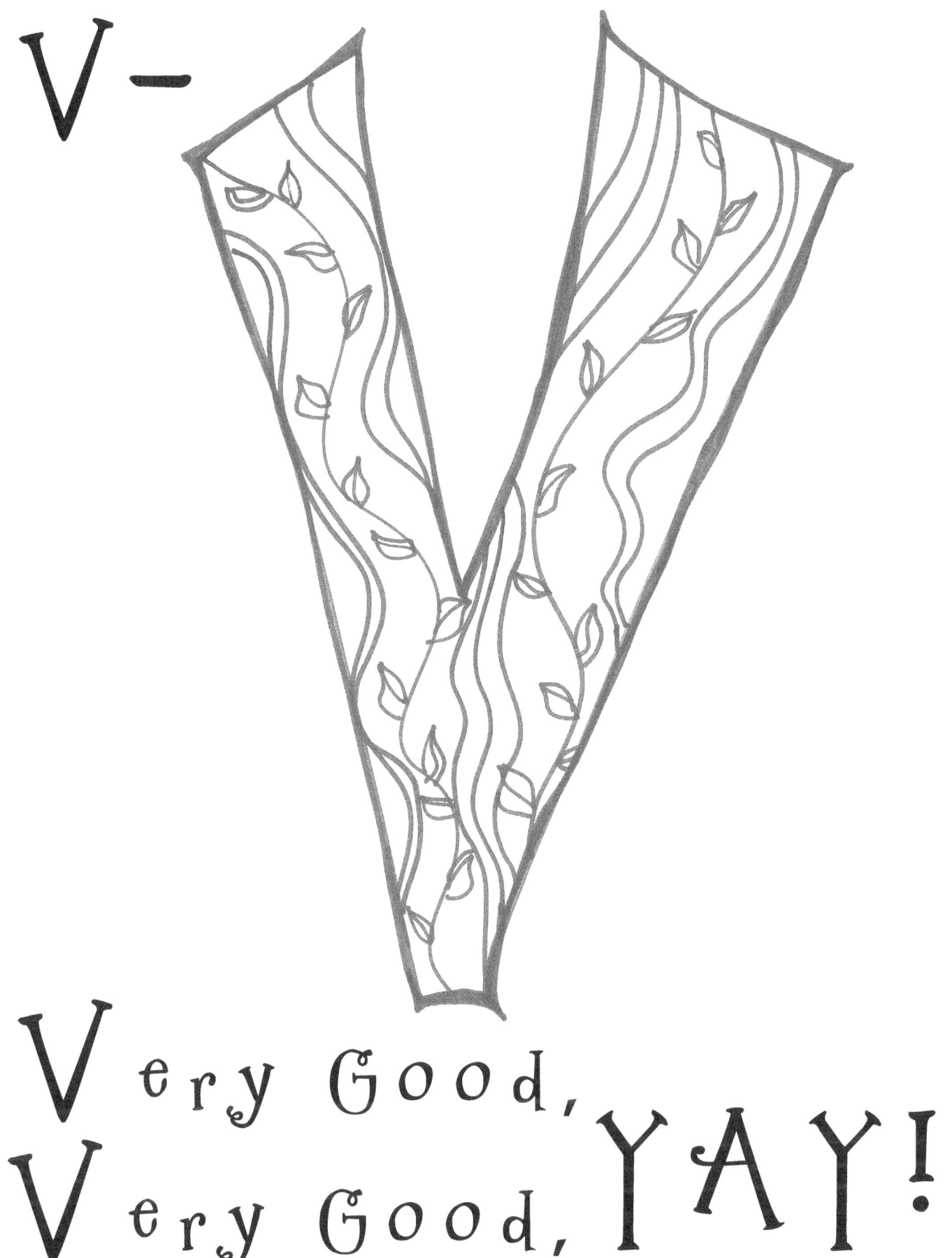

Very Good,
Very Good, YAY!

(In Laughter Yoga that's what we say!)

W-

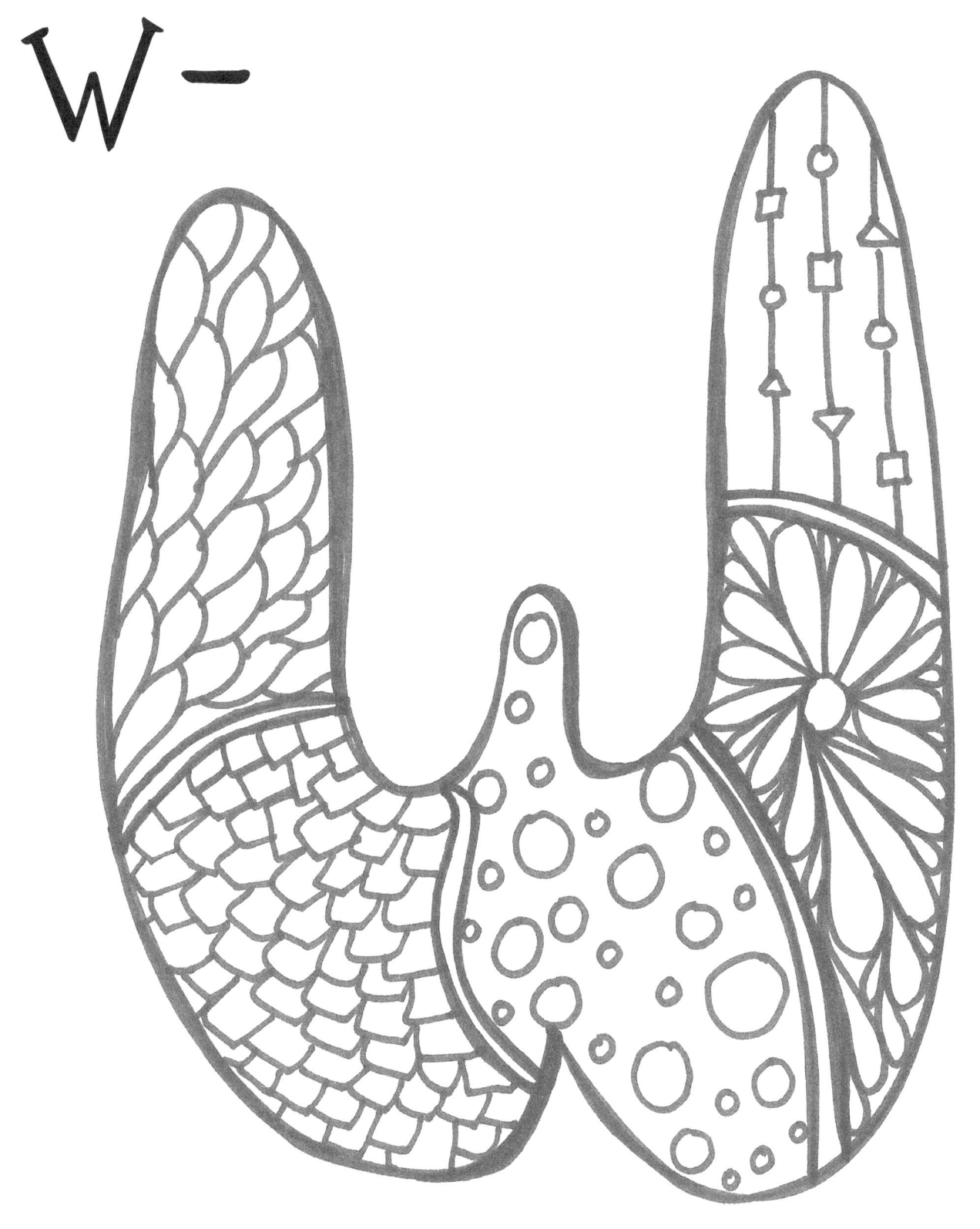

Wow! Who knew?

X-

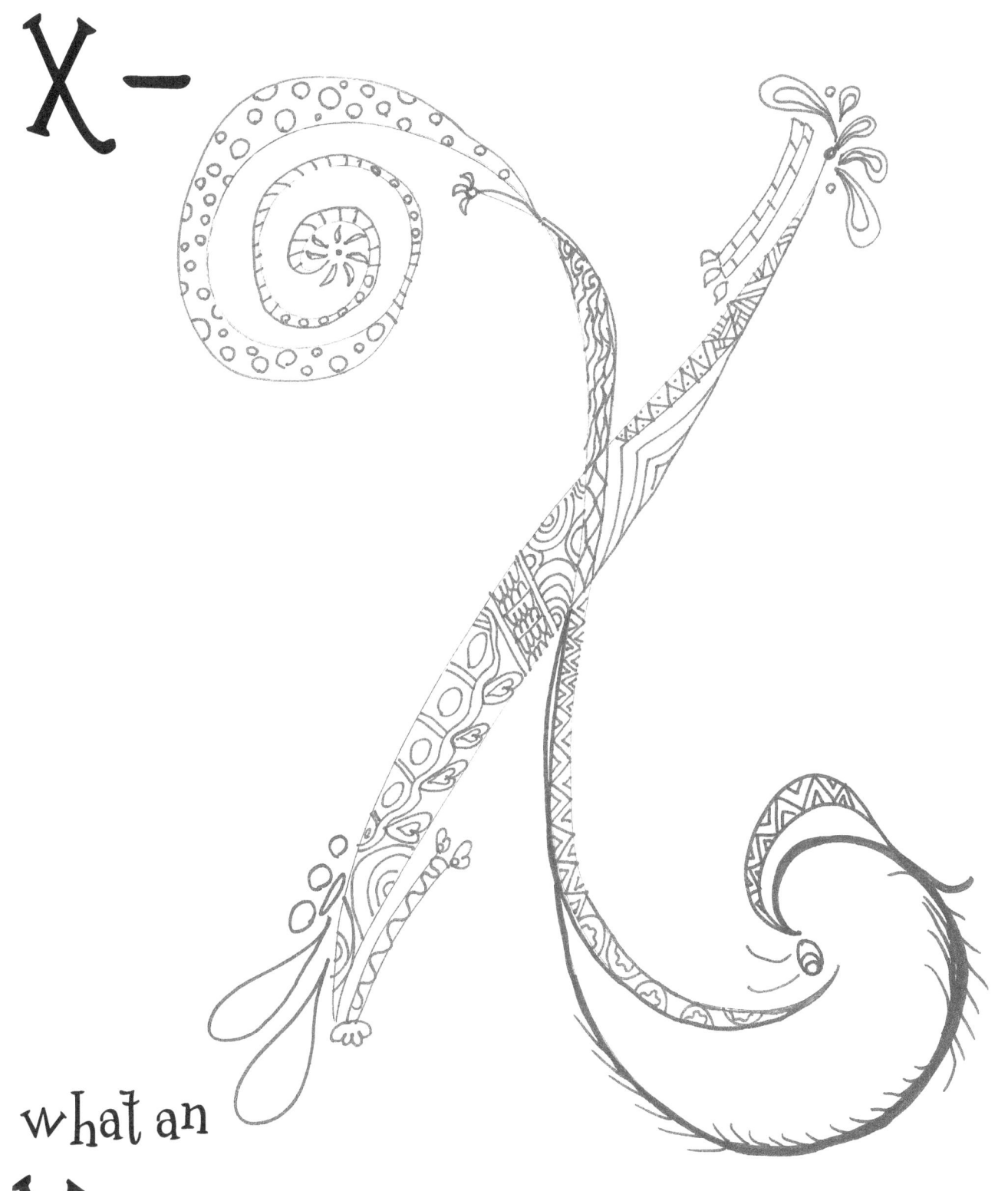

what an
Xtra-ordinary
approach to wellness!

Y-

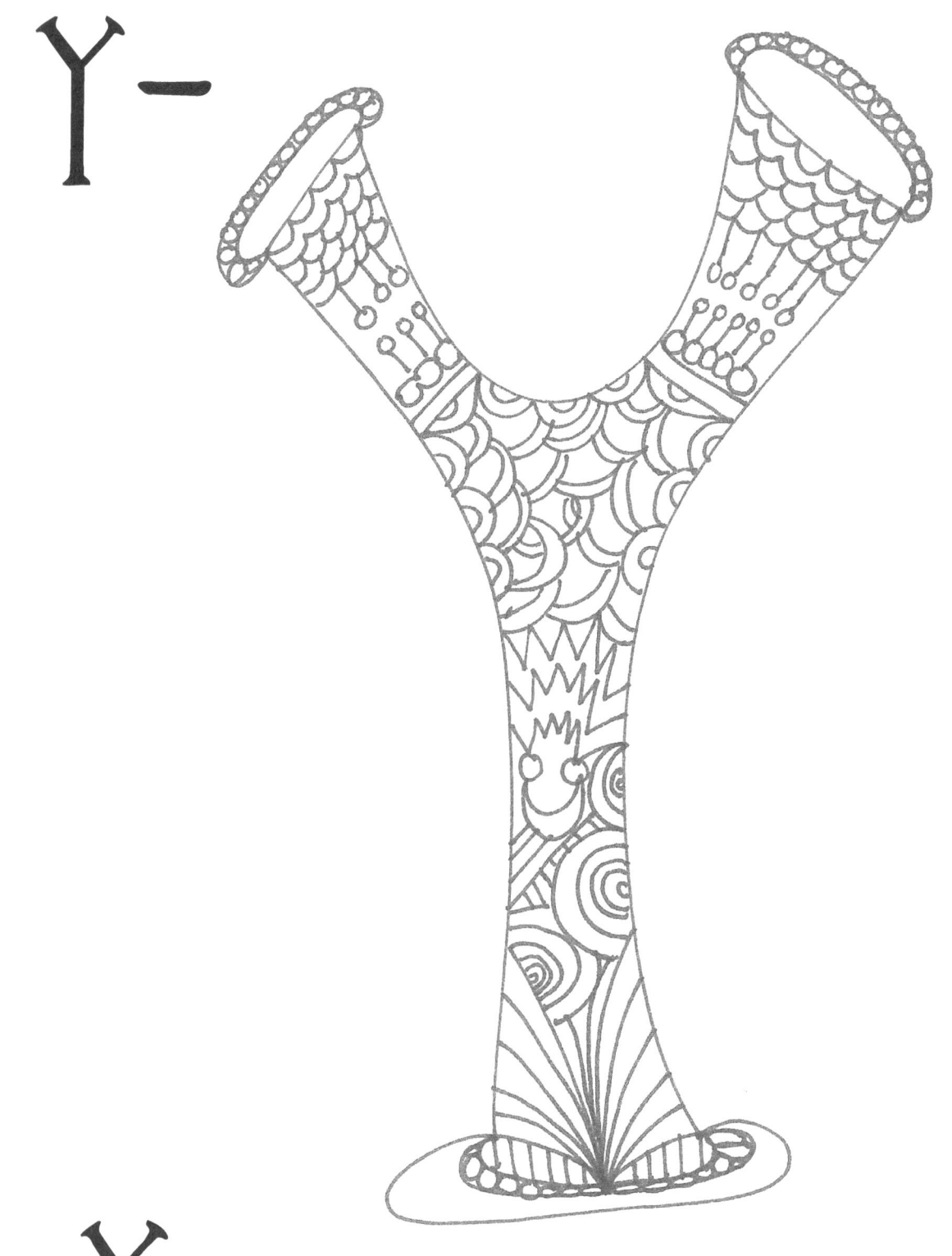

You can transform your life with laughter.

Z -

Keep a Zillio
in your pocke
better sleep!

Y–

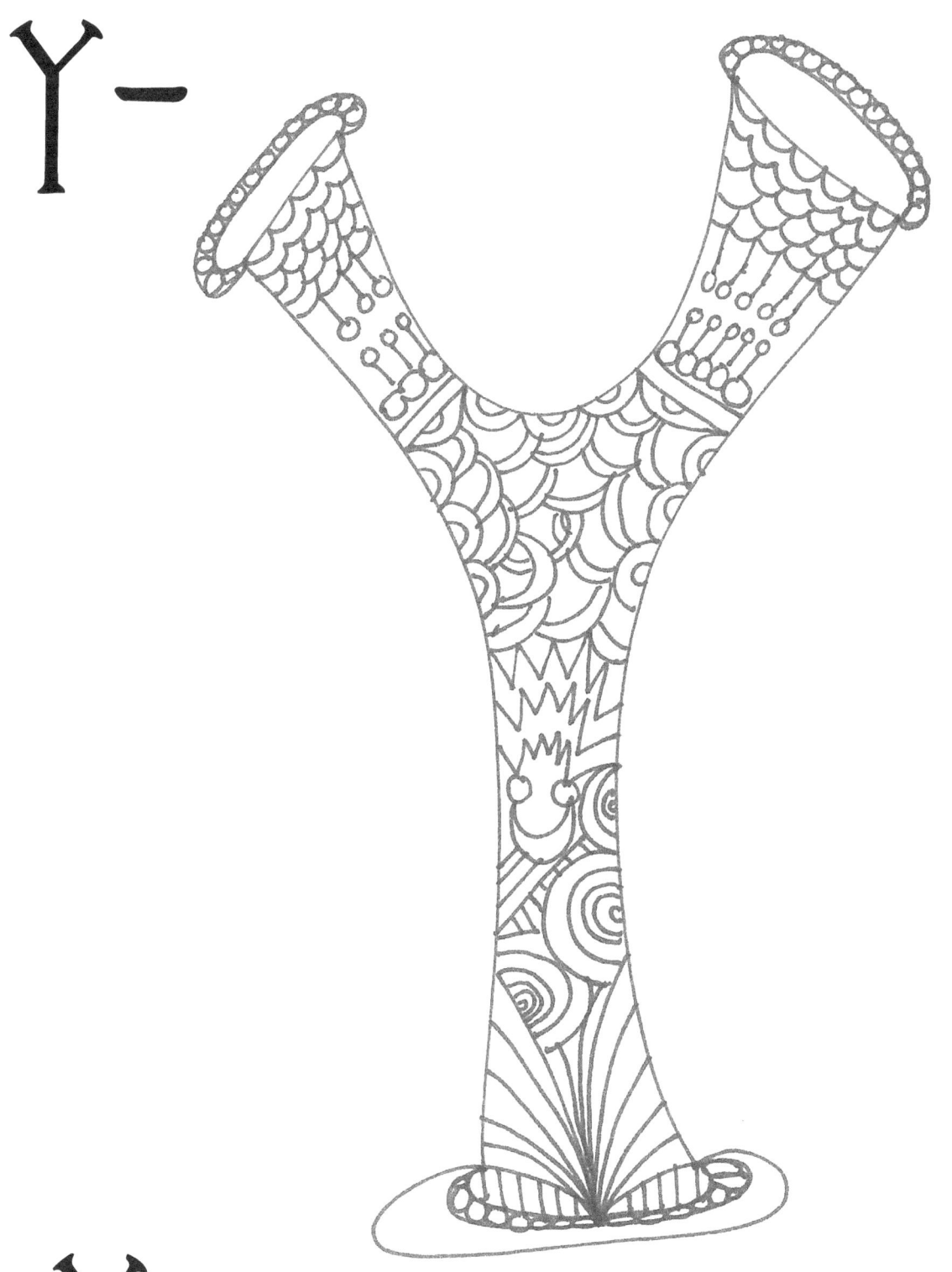

Y ou can transform
your life with laughter.

Z-

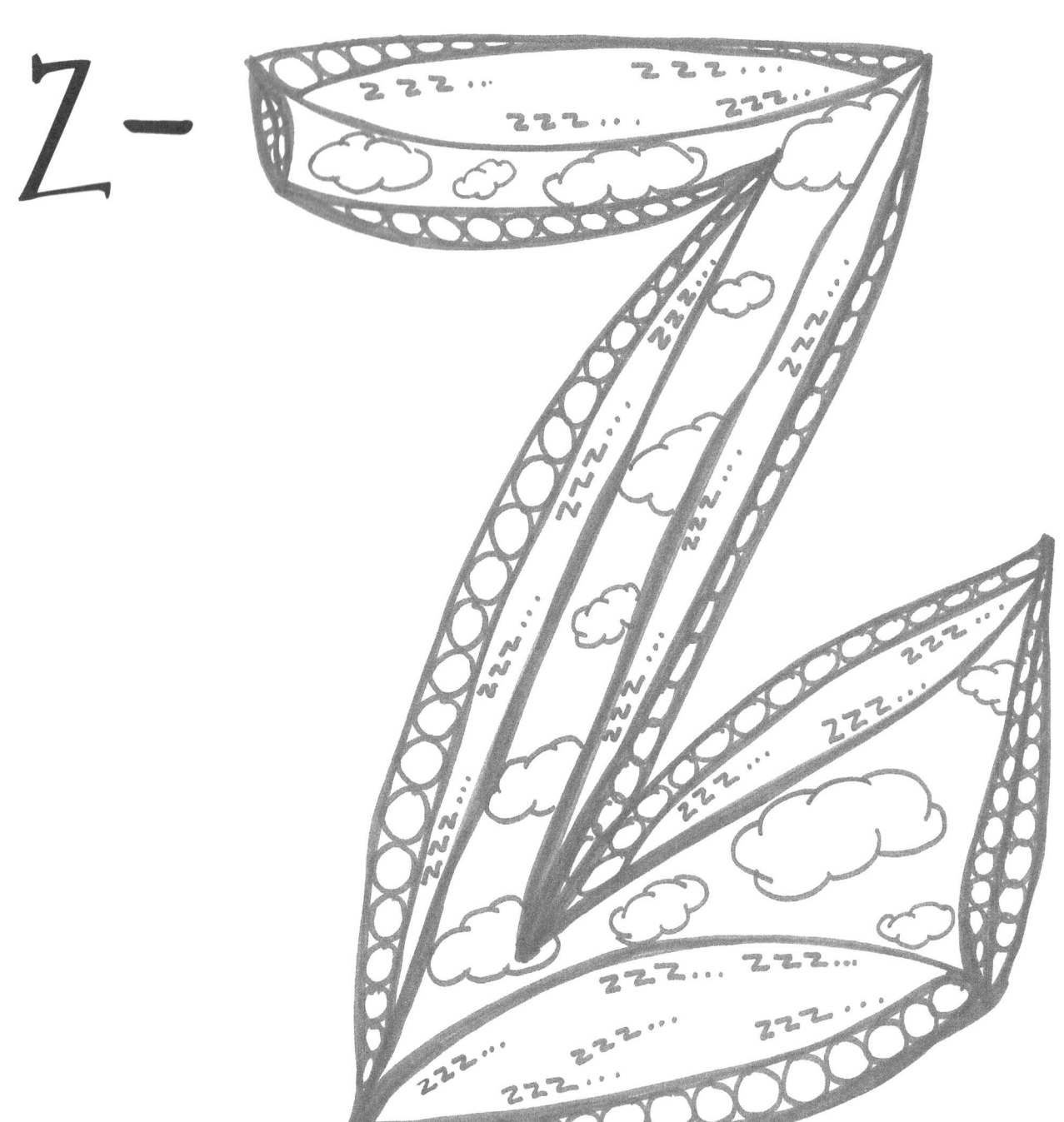

Keep a Zillion giggles in your pocket and get Letter sleep! ZZZ...